AF207032

# TEEN GUIDE:
# ADHD

by Kari A. Cornell

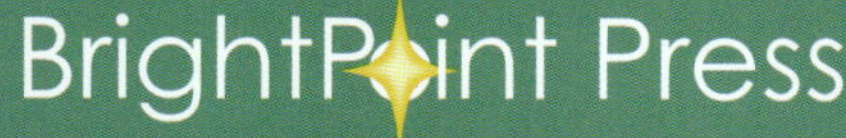

BrightPoint Press

San Diego, CA

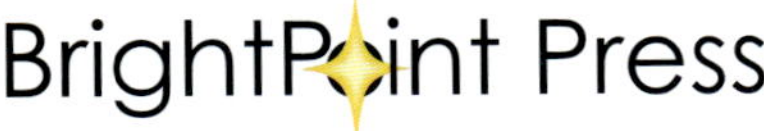


© 2026 BrightPoint Press
an imprint of ReferencePoint Press, Inc.
Printed in the United States

For more information, contact:
BrightPoint Press
PO Box 27779
San Diego, CA 92198
www.BrightPointPress.com



Content Consultant: Samantha Kempker-Margherio, Assistant Professor, Department of Psychology, Virginia Tech

LIBRARY OF CONGRESS CATALOGING-IN-PUBLICATION DATA

Names: Cornell, Kari A. author
Title: Teen guide: ADHD / by Kari A. Cornell.
Other titles: ADHD
Description: San Diego, CA: BrightPoint Press, [2026] | Series: Teen guide to mental health | Includes bibliographical references and index. | Audience: Grades 7–9
Identifiers: LCCN 2024062182 (print) | LCCN 2024062183 (eBook) | ISBN 9781678211400 hardcover | ISBN 9781678211417 (eBook)
Subjects: LCSH: Attention-deficit hyperactivity disorder in adolescence--Juvenile literature | Attention-deficit hyperactivity disorder--Juvenile literature | Youth with attention-deficit hyperactivity disorder--Juvenile literature
Classification: LCC RJ506.H9 C674 2026 (print) | LCC RJ506.H9 (eBook) | DDC 618.92/8589--dc23/eng/20250324
LC record available at https://lccn.loc.gov/2024062182
LC eBook record available at https://lccn.loc.gov/2024062183

# CONTENTS

# AT A GLANCE

- Current research suggests that ADHD affects about 11 percent of people between the ages of 3 and 17 in the United States.

- A person diagnosed with ADHD will probably always have it. But there are ways to make living with it easier.

- People with ADHD display many different symptoms. These could include trouble paying attention, hyperactivity, and impulsivity.

- Not everyone with ADHD is affected in the same way. For example, symptoms may be different for boys than for girls.

- ADHD can negatively affect someone's schoolwork and personal relationships.

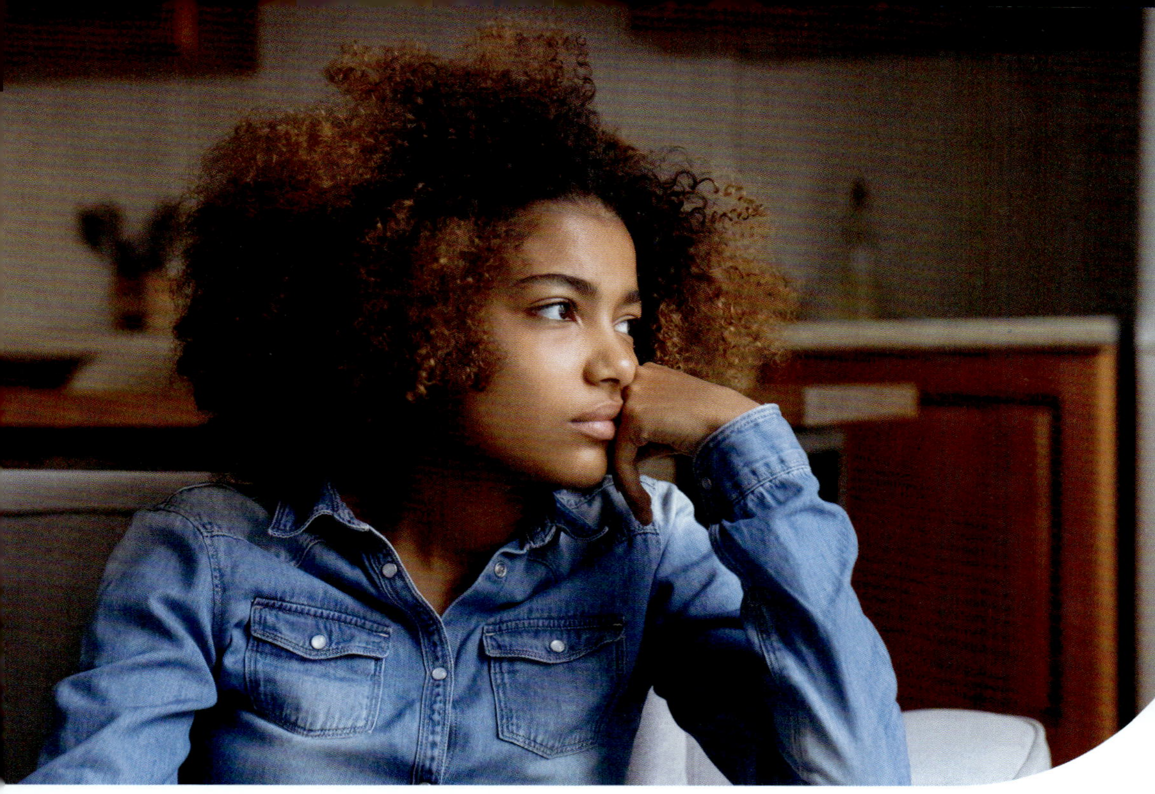

- Some people with ADHD consider some of their symptoms as strengths. These strengths include hyperfocus and having lots of energy.

- Between 1997 and 2016, ADHD diagnoses in US children and teens increased from about 6 percent to about 10 percent.

- Medication is often used with therapy to treat ADHD symptoms. This medication includes stimulants and nonstimulants.

# STRUGGLING TO FOCUS

When Morgan was in kindergarten, she had a harder time focusing than many of her peers. She struggled to do tasks that were easy for her classmates. She would quickly become distracted.

Her mother, Tina, noticed these challenges. She worked with the school to see what they could do for her daughter. The school agreed to have a **psychologist** test Morgan. She took many tests.

**Young children with ADHD often have trouble doing tasks they find boring.**

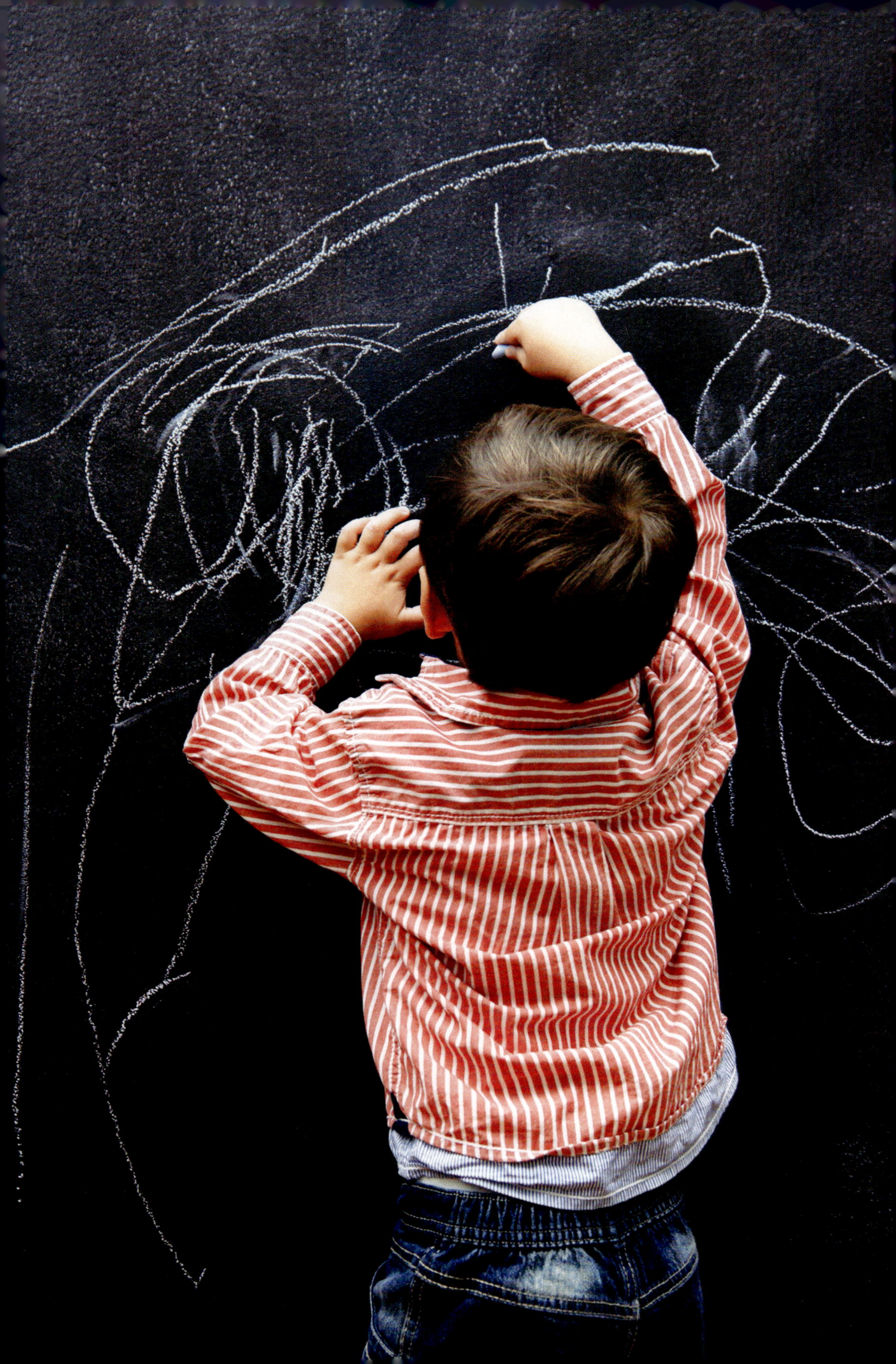

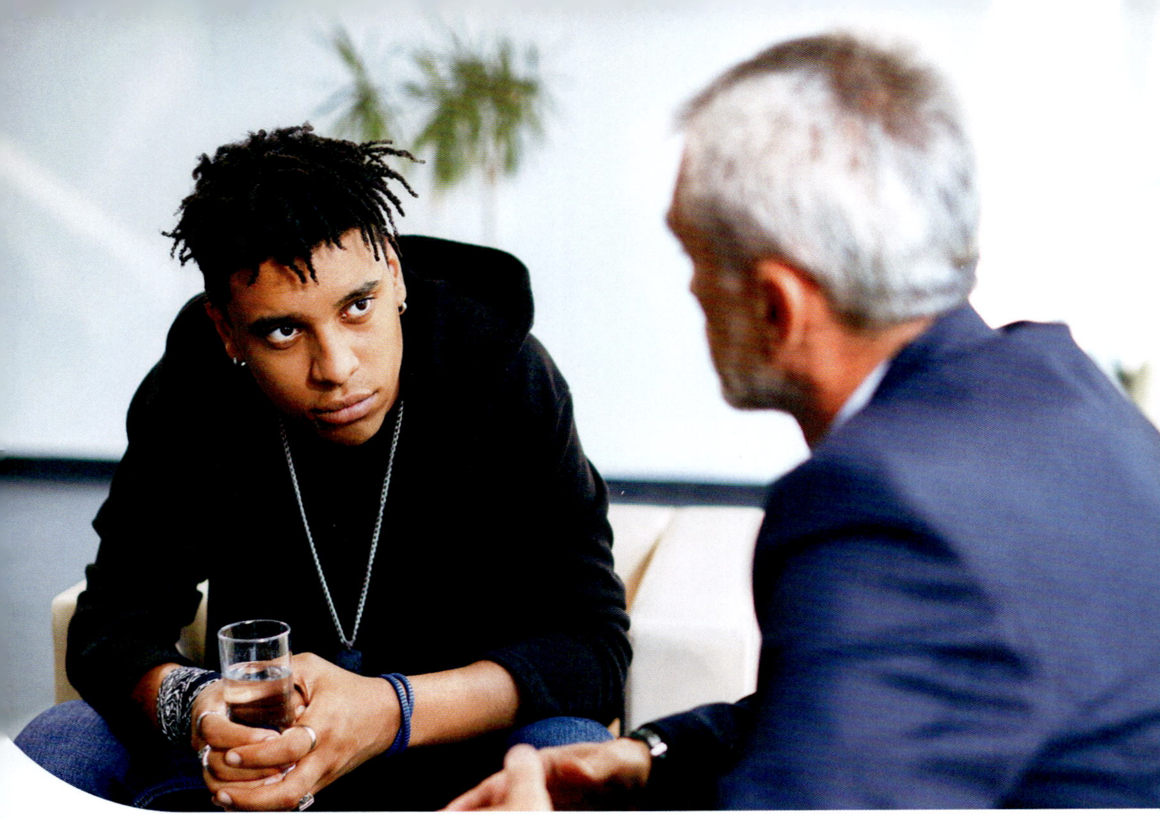



These tests helped the psychologist learn about Morgan's strengths and needs. This was how Morgan learned that she had attention deficit hyperactivity disorder (ADHD) in first grade.

Morgan grew quiet as a fourth grader. She did not talk to other kids. She did not speak up in class. Tina volunteered in Morgan's classroom. She was surprised by how her daughter acted. At home Morgan was chatty and outgoing. But at school, Morgan seemed like a different person.

The school used certain measures to try to help Morgan. Morgan recalls this time. She says,

> My first memory that things were different was when the teacher put headphones on me in the classroom. Also, things like having to go outside to a trailer classroom while my friends stayed in the regular class.[1]

Each day teachers sent home the work she had not finished. Morgan's homework piled up. She was overwhelmed.

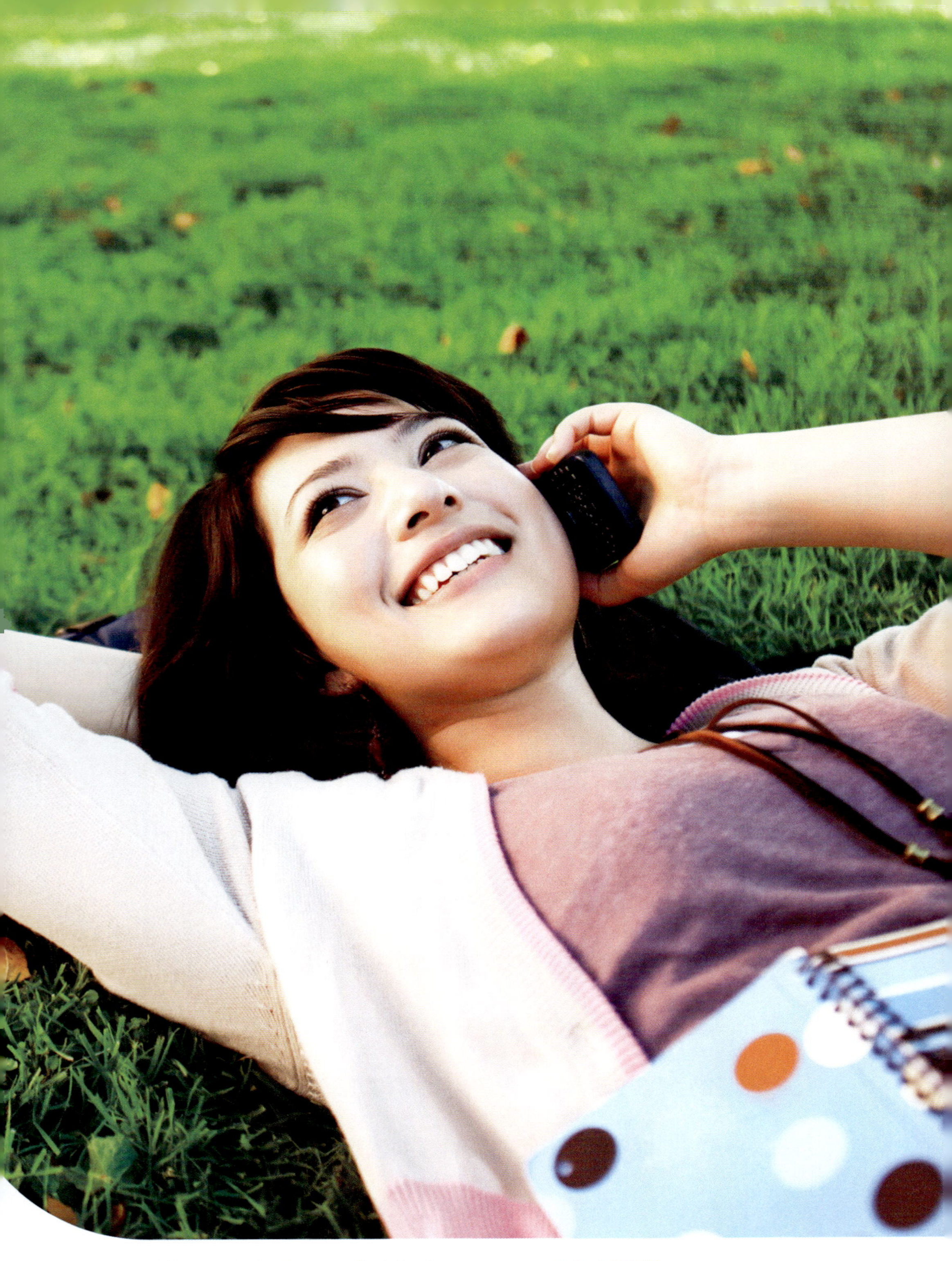

**There is help available for teens with ADHD.**

# UNDERSTANDING ADHD

Morgan was not alone. Estimates say ADHD affects about 11 percent of young people between the ages of 3 and 17 in the United States. People with ADHD have many different **symptoms**. Most have trouble focusing. They may move constantly and be easily distracted. Some fidget or tap things with their feet or fingers. People with ADHD might also make quick decisions. They may not always think before they act.

A person **diagnosed** with ADHD will probably always have it. But there are ways to make living with it easier. What may work for one person might not work for another person. The first step to managing symptoms is to learn more about this condition.

# CHAPTER ONE

# WHAT IS ADHD?

People with ADHD can have difficulty focusing. This makes it hard to learn and stay on task. Many people, including those without ADHD, sometimes struggle with focusing. But these problems are more severe for those with ADHD. They also happen more often. And these challenges can negatively affect their schoolwork or career.

**Teens with ADHD who struggle to complete their homework may need support from parents and teachers.**

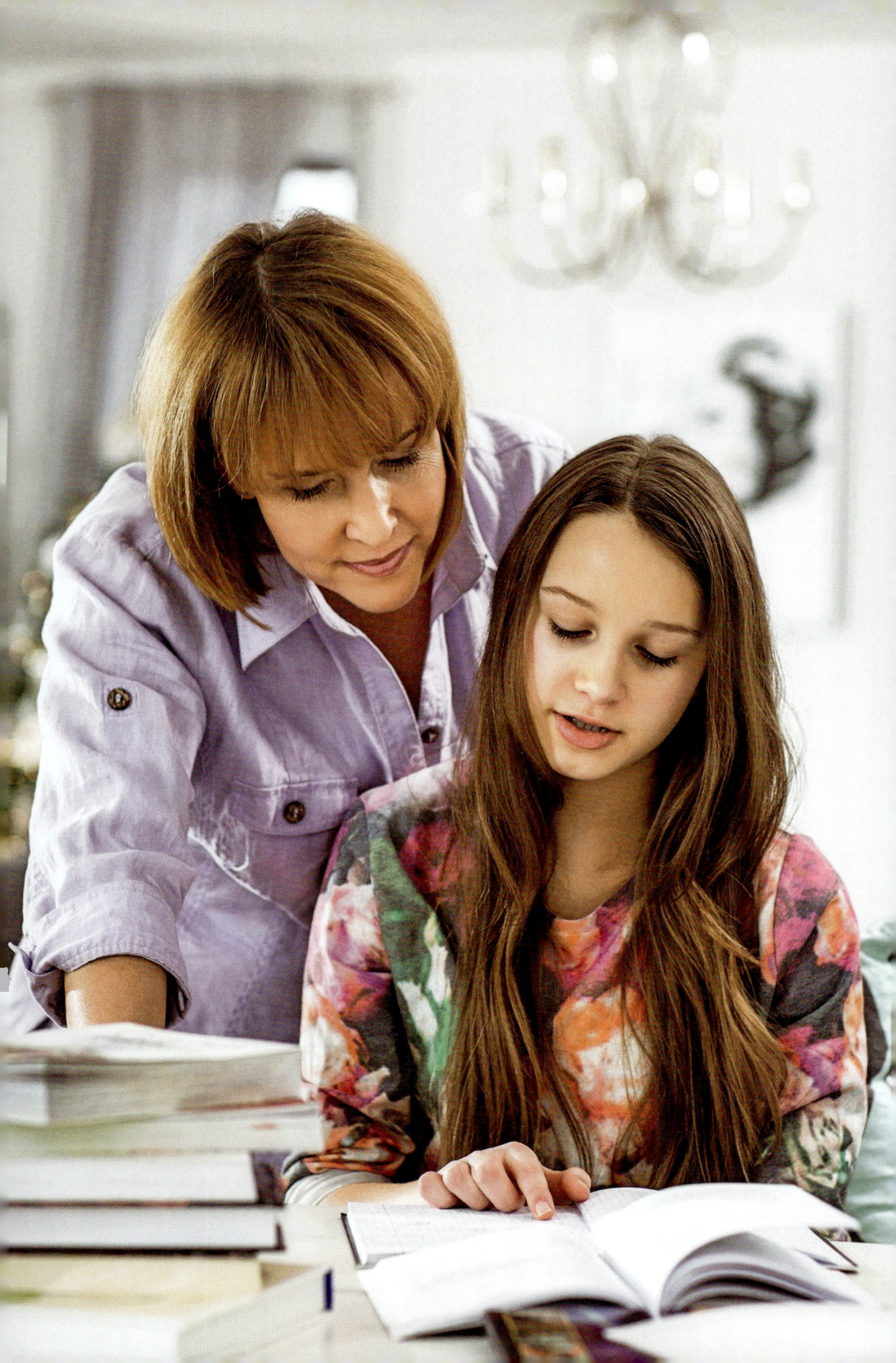

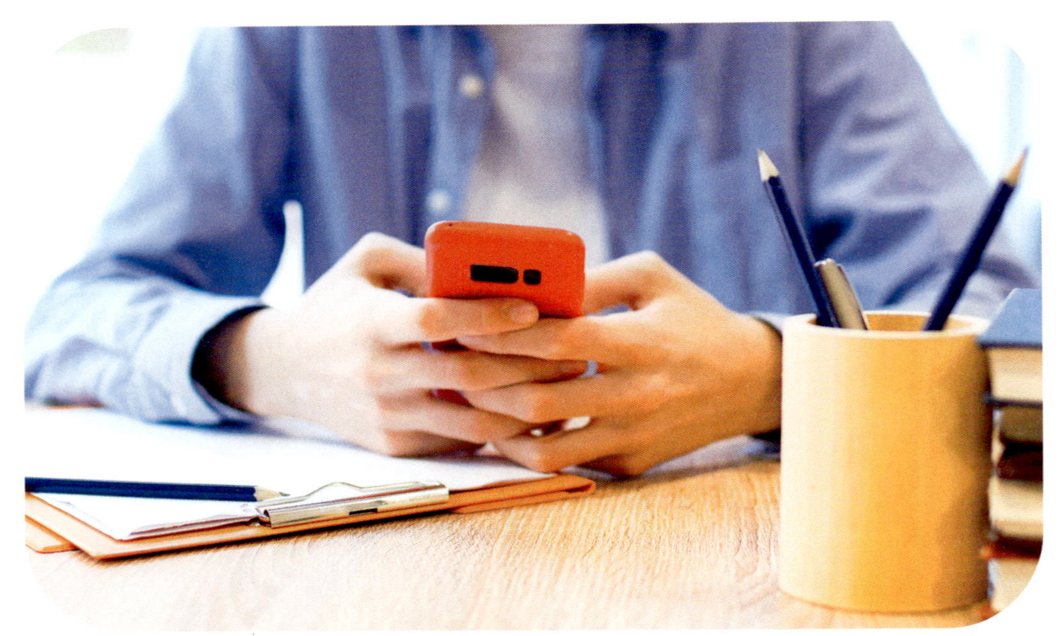



Judee is a teen with ADHD. She says, "Having ADHD is like having a billion trampolines in your head . . . and your brain [is] just jumping off each and every one every second."[2] This is what daily life is like for many teens with ADHD.

## SYMPTOMS OF ADHD

ADHD has a long list of symptoms. But not everyone with ADHD is affected in the same way. Symptoms may be different for boys and girls. And some symptoms can fade as a person with ADHD grows older.

Many people first learn that they have ADHD in school. Schools often require students to sit and pay attention for long periods of time. This can be difficult for people who experience hyperactivity as part of their ADHD. Hyperactivity is the state of being more active than is appropriate for a given situation.

Hyperactivity affects many classroom tasks and skills. Kids with ADHD often have a hard time sitting still. They may be easily distracted. They may also have trouble listening. Focusing on lessons in class can be difficult. Students with ADHD often have trouble finishing homework. They may forget to hand in assignments. They may also lack patience. Sometimes they rush through tasks to finish them. This can lead to errors.

Other symptoms of ADHD relate to organization. People with ADHD may be absent-minded. They may be disorganized. This can cause them to lose things often. Or they might forget scheduled events such as appointments. Some with ADHD may need constant reminders to keep commitments.

Impulsivity is another common symptom of ADHD. It causes people to act without thinking. Impulsivity can cause a person to interrupt others. People with impulsivity may do unsafe things even when they know know it is dangerous. Teens with ADHD may be more likely to try risky behaviors.

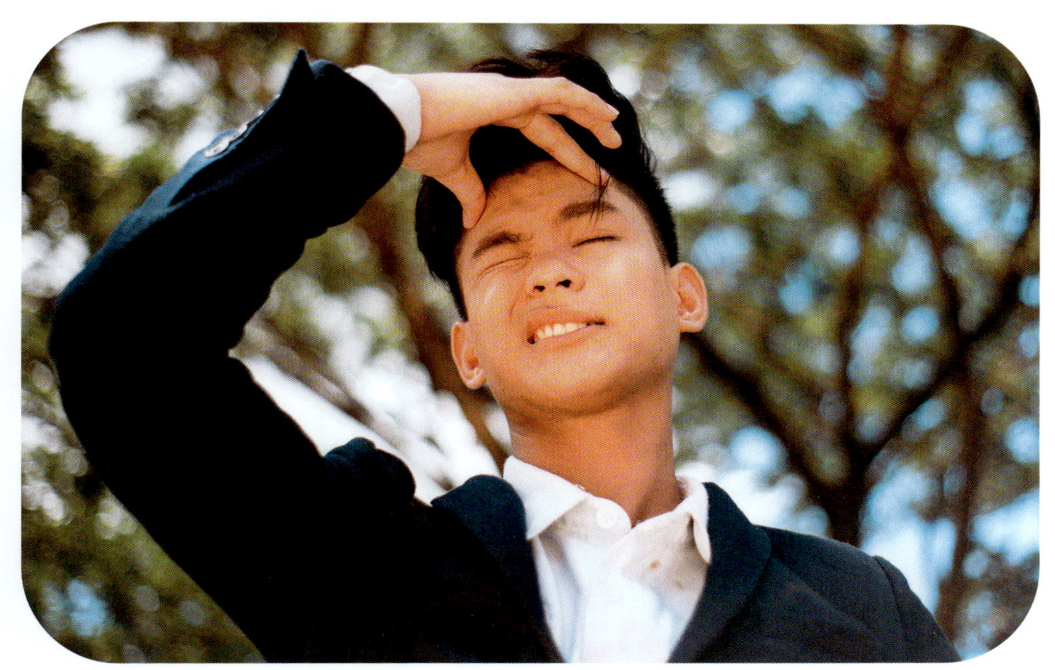

**Teens with ADHD may have trouble being on time. Researchers are studying how ADHD can affect a person's perception of time.**

These behaviors can include unsafe substance use and unsafe sexual activity.

Some with ADHD also struggle with emotion dysregulation (ED). This is when people have trouble controlling their emotions. Their reactions to events may seem outsized. And it may take longer than typical for them to calm down. ED can

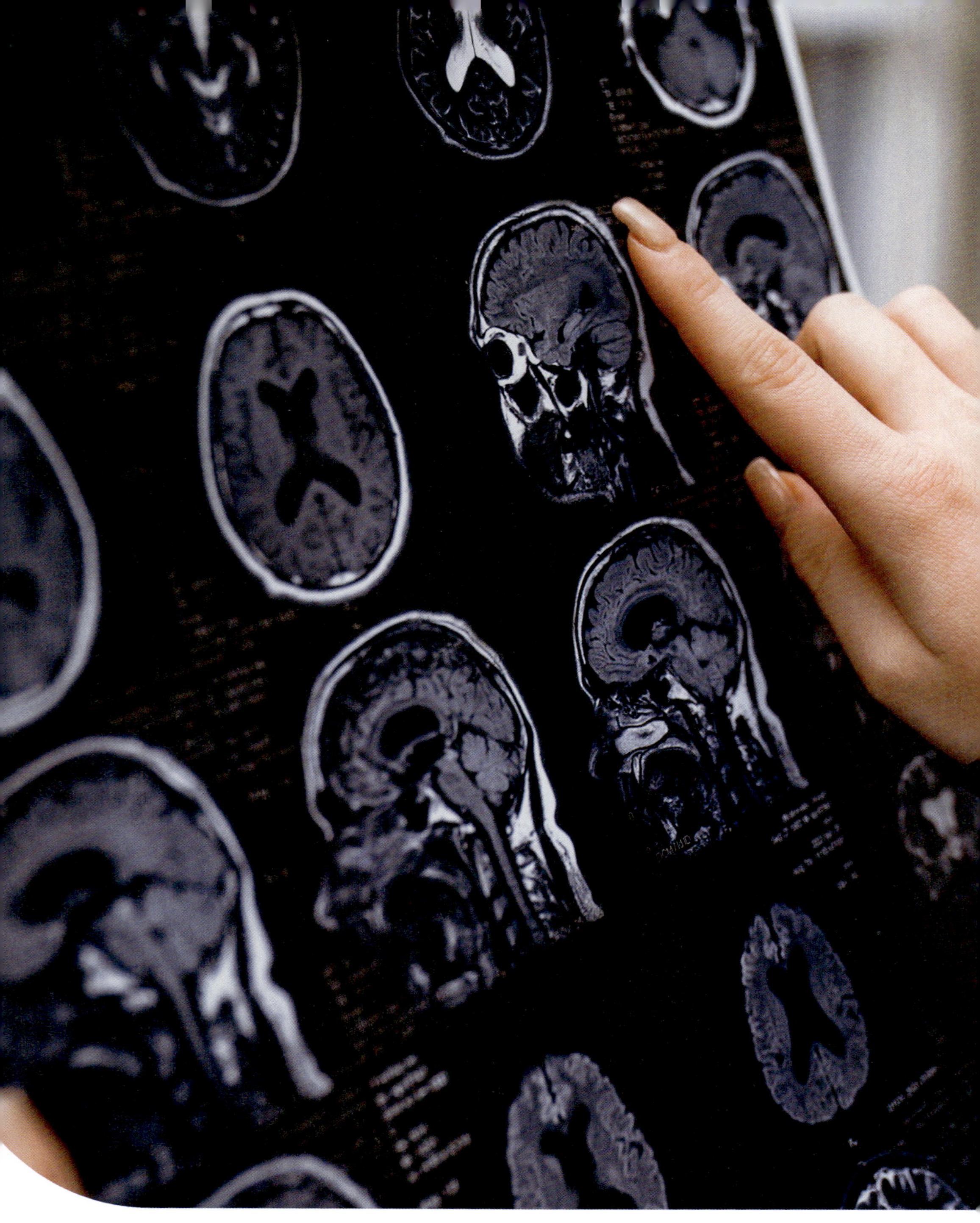

Researchers can study the structures of people's brains using scans made with medical imaging equipment.

affect people's negative and positive emotions. People with ED may have trouble controlling feelings of sadness or anger. They may also have trouble controlling excitement. Researchers are studying the connection between ADHD and ED. One aim is to find treatments that help people with ADHD control ED.

## DIFFERENCES IN BRAIN STRUCTURE

Studies show that people with ADHD may have a smaller prefrontal cortex. This part of the brain allows people to make decisions. It also regulates emotions.

The basal ganglia may also be smaller in people with ADHD. Basal ganglia are a cluster of cells near the center of the brain.

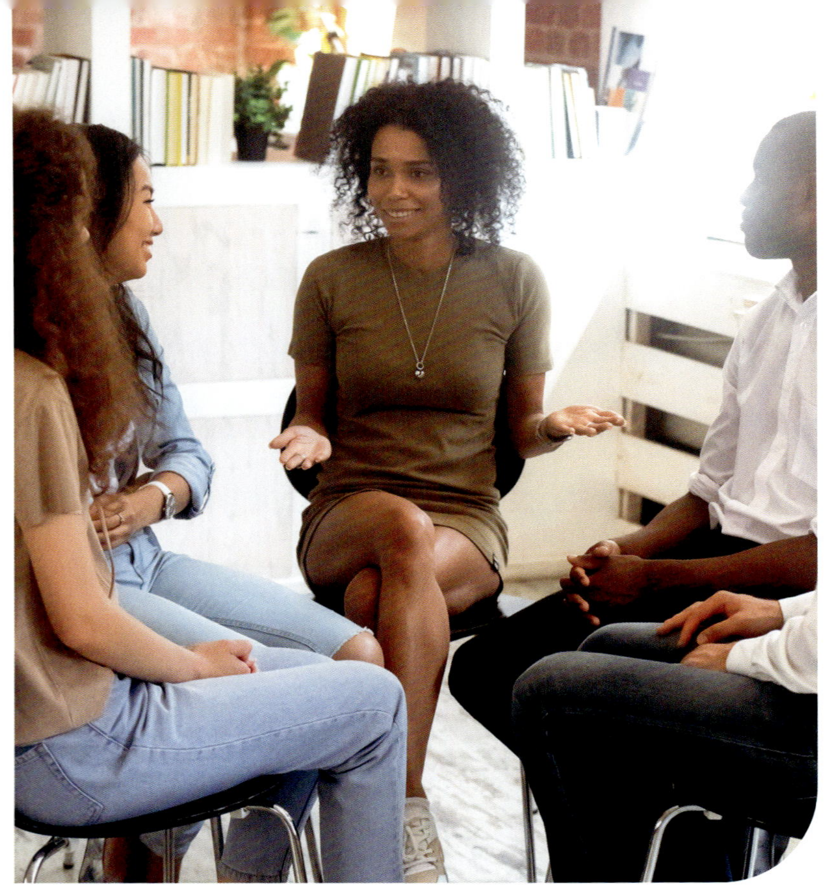

Studying people's reactions in controlled situations is one way that psychologists learn about the human mind.

They form connections between different parts of the brain. These cells are part of a network of nerves that help control the body's movement. Basal ganglia also help the brain consider risks and set goals. And they aid in processing emotions. They also help with completing tasks. This means

the basal ganglia are key to learning.
These functions can be difficult for those
with ADHD.

Another study gave people a difficult
problem to think through. Some had
ADHD, while others did not. Both groups
had a hard time solving the problem. But
researchers noticed something. The anterior
cingulate cortex was not active in those with
ADHD. This part of the brain helps people
control what they focus on. It was very
active in those without ADHD.

Instead, those with ADHD relied on the
brain's default mode network (DMN). This
network takes over when other regions
of the brain are resting. The DMN works
when people are not doing specific tasks.
It allows a person to continue thinking

behind the scenes. For example, the DMN is responsible for daydreaming.

The DMN is not always active in a person who does not have ADHD. It stops working when other parts of the brain step in to



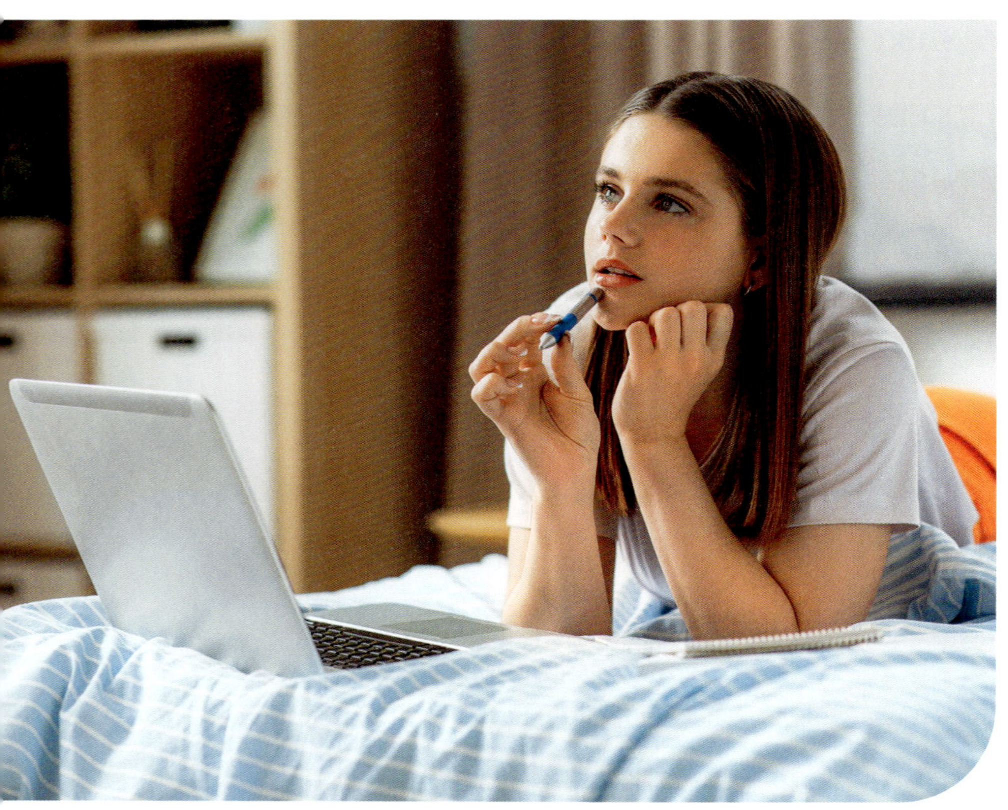

complete tasks. But the DMN never stops working in a person with ADHD. This may explain why those with ADHD often seem to be thinking of other things. An overactive DMN may contribute to their distraction.

## DIAGNOSING ADHD

Many people with ADHD are diagnosed before age 12. But others may be diagnosed as teens or adults. ADHD symptoms typically continue into adulthood. Up to 90 percent of adults who were diagnosed with ADHD as children continue to have symptoms.

To diagnose ADHD, a medical doctor, psychologist, or counselor will ask a patient questions. They may also ask patients to fill out a checklist. Parents or teachers may

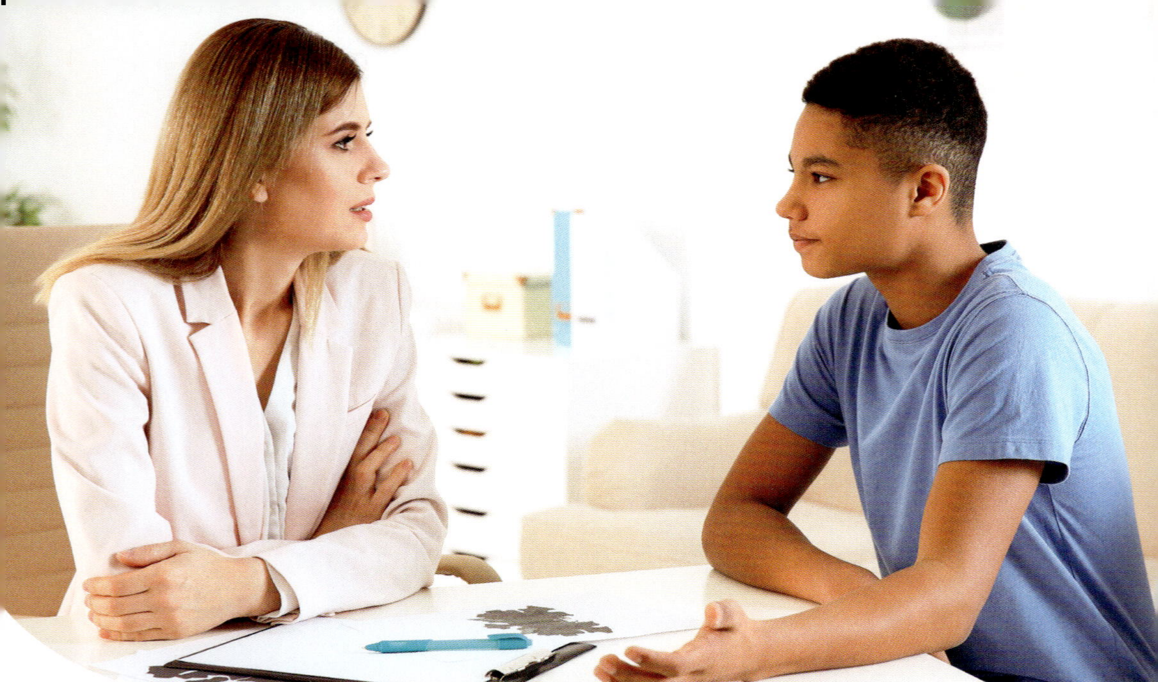



fill one out as well. The checklist contains a series of common symptoms of ADHD.

Those who are diagnosed with ADHD may have one of three types. The first is inattentive ADHD. This means most symptoms are related to an inability to focus. The second is hyperactive-impulsive ADHD. A person with this type of ADHD has symptoms related to hyperactivity and acts impulsively. The third type of ADHD

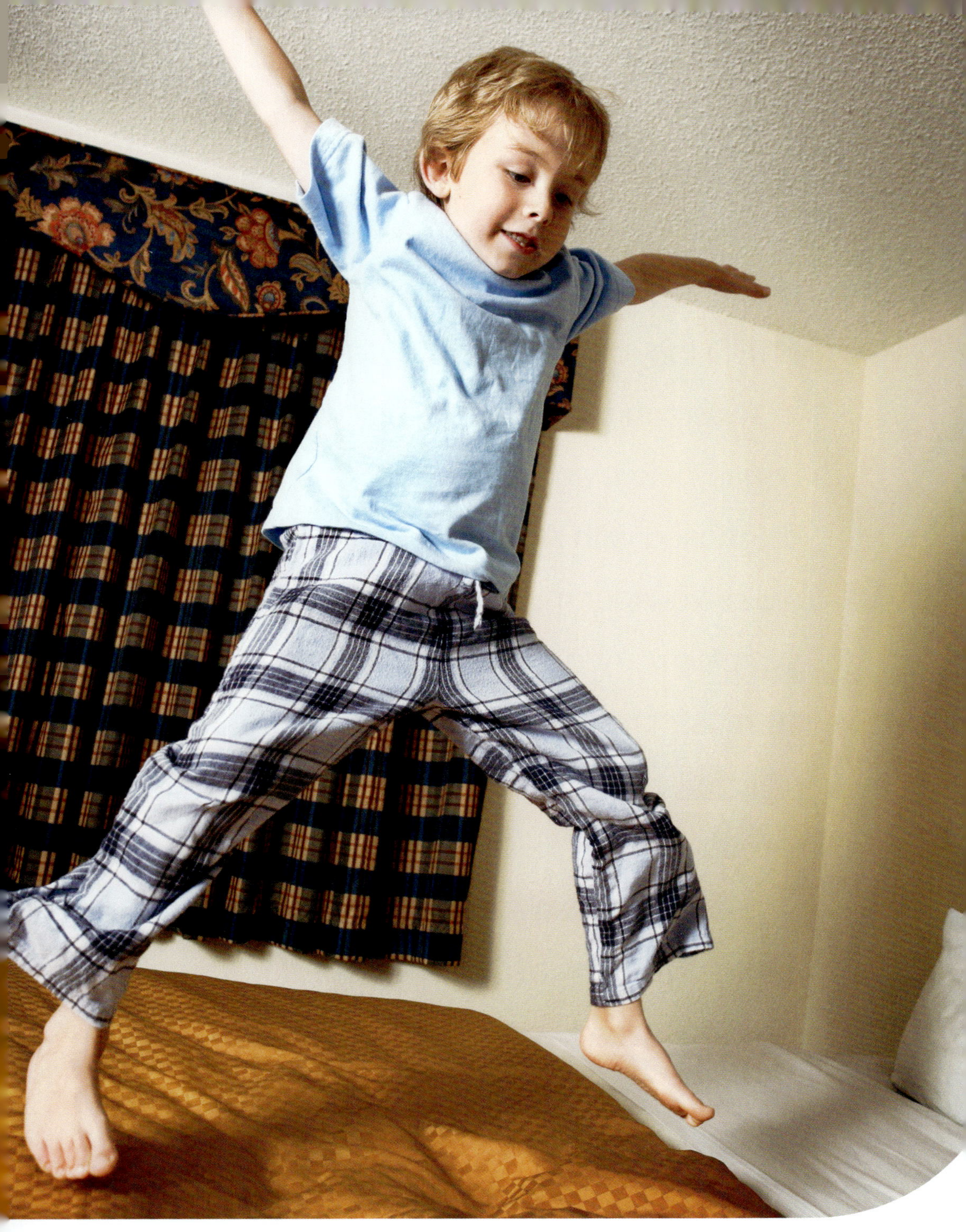

Hyperactive-impulsive ADHD is the least common type
of the condition.

is called combined. This type includes all symptoms. For many people, the type of ADHD they have will shift over time.

A person must have symptoms that began before age 12 in order to be diagnosed with ADHD. People 16 years old or younger must have six or more symptoms. And those older than 16 must have five or more symptoms.

## Coexisting Conditions

Almost 78 percent of people between 12 and 17 years old with ADHD experience other mental health conditions. About 43 percent have anxiety. More than a quarter have depression. And almost 13 percent have autism spectrum disorder. About half of youth with ADHD also experience some form of specific learning disability. Many struggle with reading.

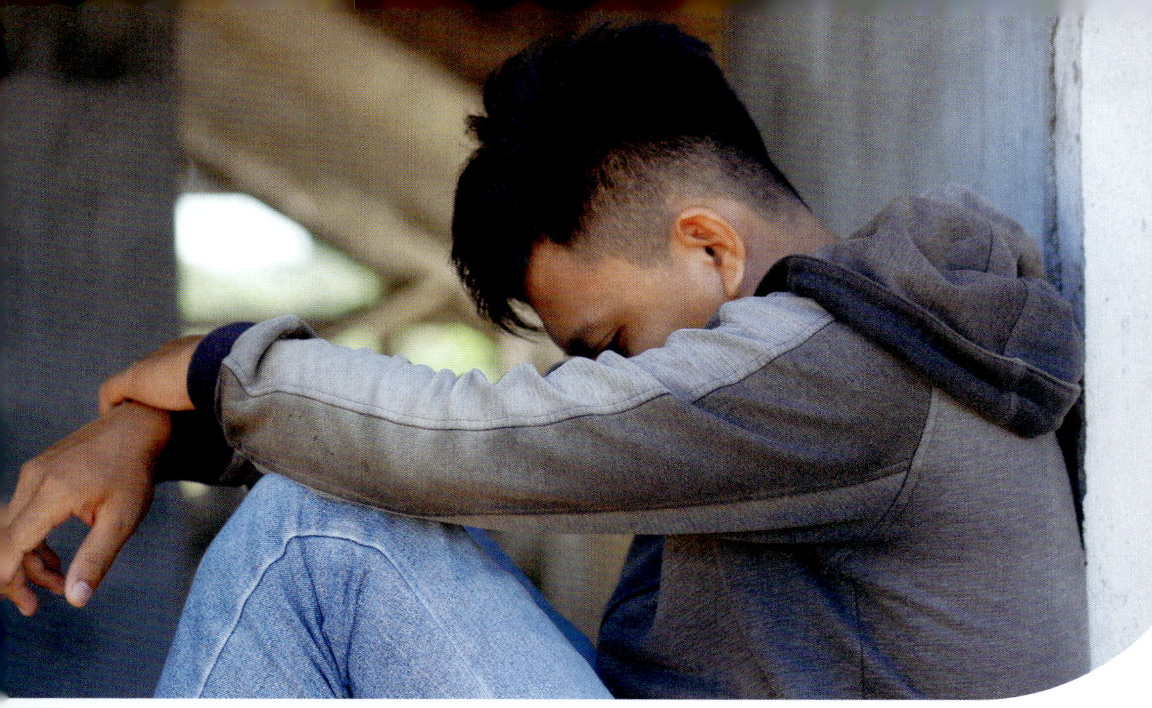



Symptoms must affect the person for at least 6 months. ADHD symptoms must also exist in two or more areas of the person's life. These areas include school, home, work, and social settings. And the symptoms must negatively affect the person's schooling, work, or ability to interact with others.

# CHAPTER TWO

# LIVING WITH ADHD

ADHD affects the lives of teens in many ways. Some mention knowing that others view them as different. Teens may also worry that people think they use their diagnosis as an excuse. And many wish they could simply sit down and do their homework without getting distracted. Living with ADHD affects everything for Josh. He says, "My ADHD affects every aspect of my life, from sleep to school to work, and all of

**Teens with ADHD may have trouble sleeping.**

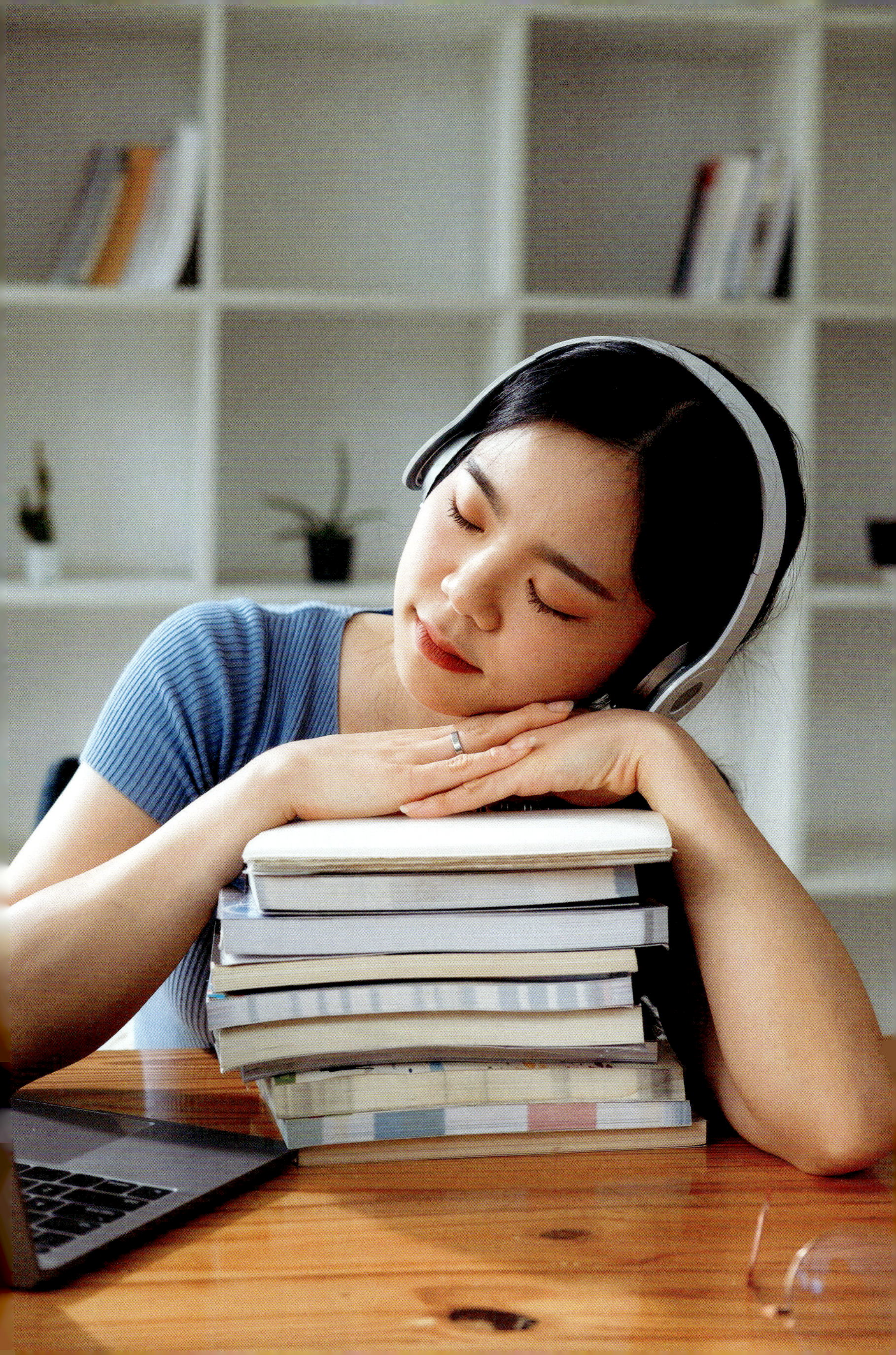

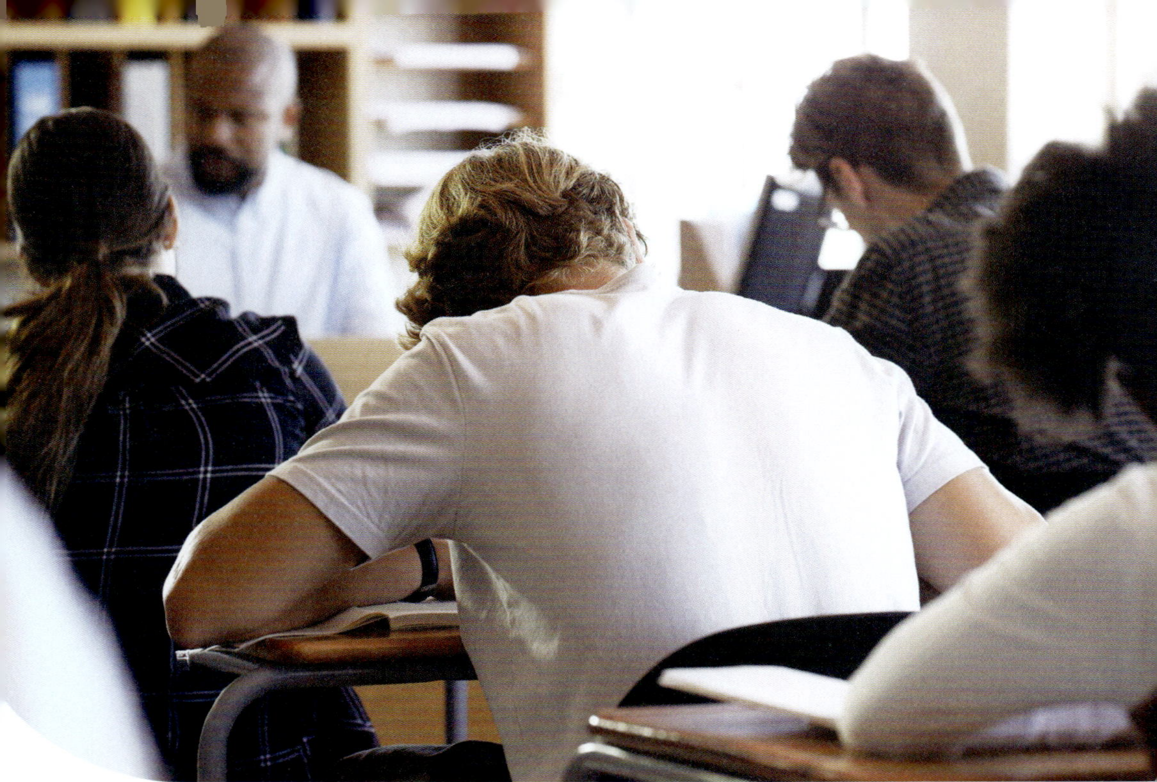



my relationships. I have to tailor my entire life around having it."[3]

Many teens find that ADHD is especially tough to manage at school. Upper grades can come with additional challenges. There are more demands on attention and organization. Task planning is another challenge. These challenges come from having multiple courses and several teachers. More independence can also cause these challenges. Dylan did well in elementary school and middle school. He got As and Bs. His teachers considered him bright. But his undiagnosed ADHD made high school difficult. His grades dropped to Cs and Ds.

Dylan explains that he struggled to balance his time. He had trouble planning activities in the future. And he could not focus on a task for long. Reading often made him fall asleep. His eyes would get tired when studying chemistry. Soon he would grow bored. He would stop and play a video game.

Dylan is not alone. Homework difficulties are common for those with ADHD. For Natalie, turning in homework on time was a challenge. Late assignments led to lower grades. Others describe how the battle to do homework affects their **self-esteem**. Kate described her frustration at not being able to do simple tasks. There were times when this made her feel unintelligent.

Ash always had trouble getting homework done. He had been fidgety since he was 4 years old. He tested well but never finished his homework. And he had trouble

## ADHD and Gender

ADHD often goes undiagnosed in girls. This may be because symptoms in girls tend not to show as much as symptoms in boys. Girls with ADHD may have low self-esteem. They may withdraw socially. Some bottle up their frustration and anger. This can lead to depression and anxiety.

controlling his daydreams. One teacher
gave him detention every day for 2 years.

## SOCIAL EFFECTS OF ADHD

ADHD can also affect relationships. Some
people with ADHD talk about having trouble
making friends. ADHD symptoms may
lead to misunderstandings. Josh explains,
"The worst part is when my symptoms
aren't taken as symptoms, they're taken
as behaviors, done intentionally to upset
someone . . . and that's never been
the case."[4]

Symptoms such as impulsivity can lead
to hurt feelings. Author Zoe Kessler's ADHD
used to cause social struggles. She says,

*Throughout my teen years, countless*

*times I made friends, only to watch the*

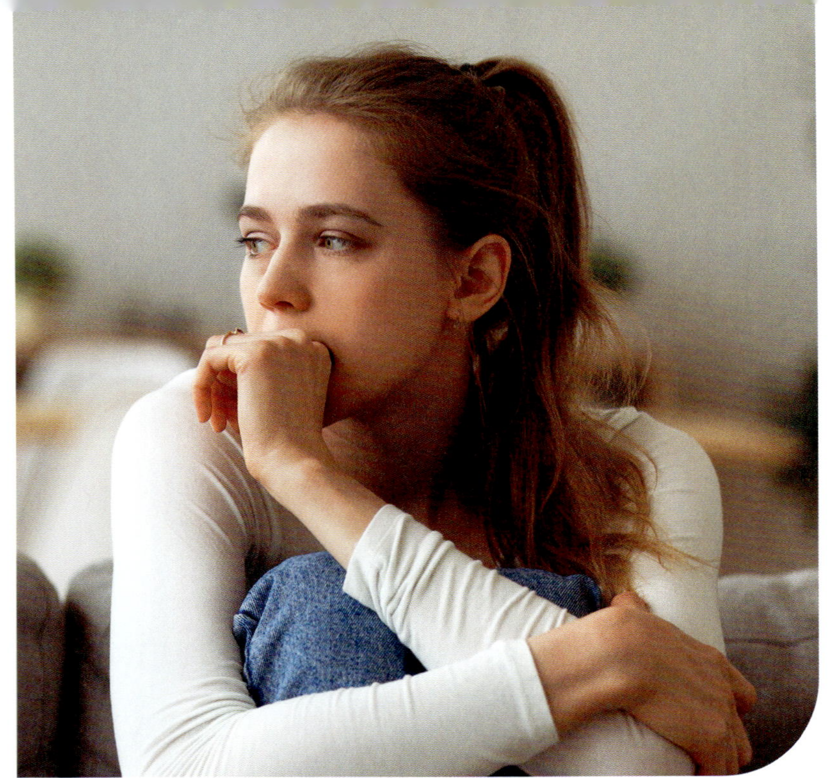

Research has shown that teens with ADHD are more likely to report feeling lonely than teens without ADHD.

friendship blow up in my face from an impulsive, careless remark. I'd be just as shocked as the friend . . . but the damage was done.[5]

Kessler also talks about feeling as if she were alone in the world. She felt different from others. Dylan felt this way as well as his ADHD worsened. He says,

*My relationships changed too. I
grew apart from old friends and
was not able to make new ones.
I viewed myself as a loner . . . .
My confidence was slipping, and I had
begun to experience the awful taste
of depression.*[6]

Research has connected ADHD with bullying. Students with ADHD are more likely to be victims of bullying than students without ADHD. Some might be bullied for their ADHD symptoms These include hyperactivity and impulsivity. Students with ADHD are also more likely to be bullies than students without ADHD. Frustration with their ADHD symptoms may cause some students to take out their anger on others.

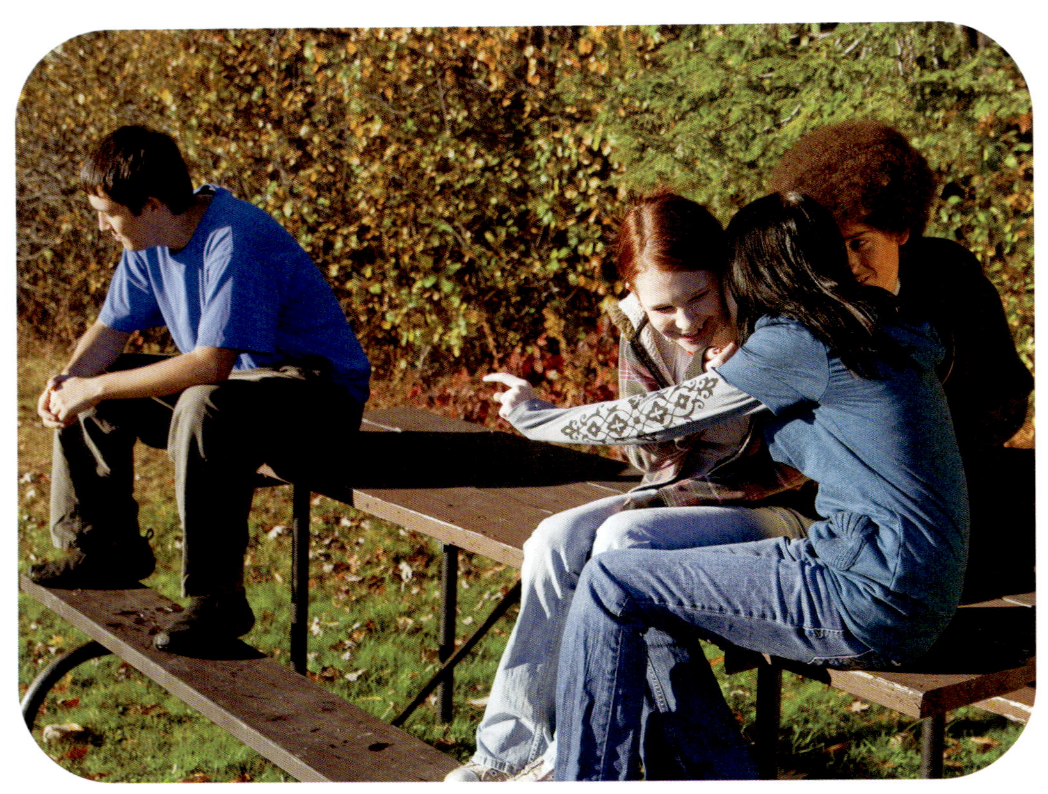

A 2019 study found that one out of every five students has been bullied.

But not all relationship experiences are negative ones for those with ADHD. Ash tells the story of meeting Cheyenne. Cheyenne had ADHD. Ash listened to her talk about her symptoms. This was how he realized he might have ADHD too. Like Ash, Cheyenne had trouble finishing schoolwork. She talked quickly. She jumped from topic to topic. But Ash had no problem following the conversation. It felt normal. He felt a sense of connection with Cheyenne. It made him feel less alone.

## STRENGTHS OF ADHD

Some people with ADHD find benefits in their symptoms. Many people with ADHD

**Meeting other people with ADHD can help teens cope with having the condition.**

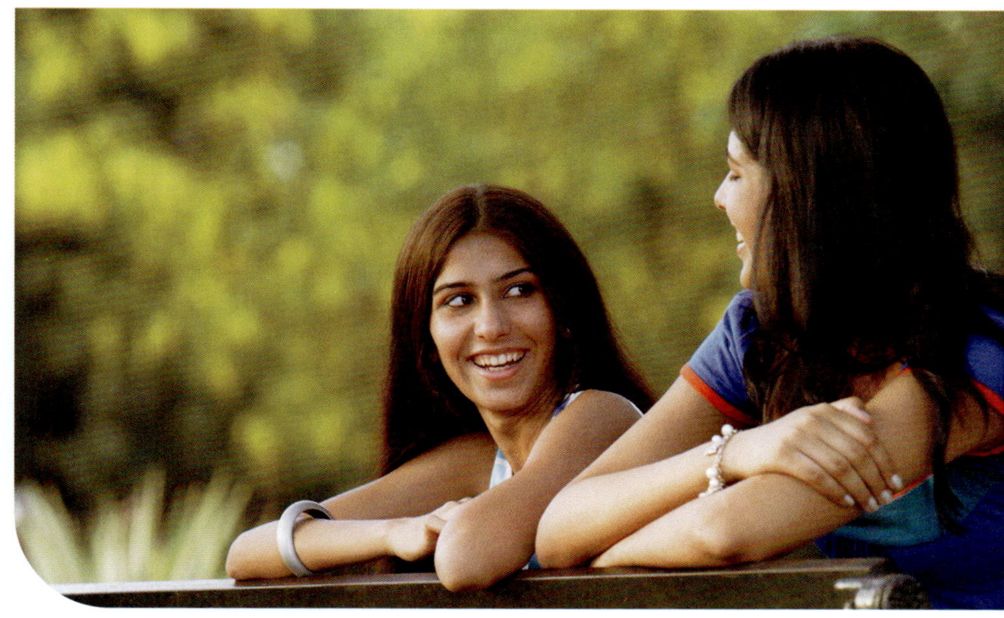

report experiencing hyperfocus. This produces a state of deep concentration. It allows people to work on a project for hours at a time.

Alisa Cheng remembers her first moment of hyperfocus. She was diagnosed with ADHD at 15. She began taking **medication** to help her focus. But she did not know how to stay focused.

One day, Alisa signed up for an international contest. It was a test on ophthalmology. This is the field of medicine that treats eye problems. She admits she was often distracted as she studied. She watched a lot of unrelated YouTube videos. But she also opened several articles on ophthalmology. She would glance at the articles between videos. She became

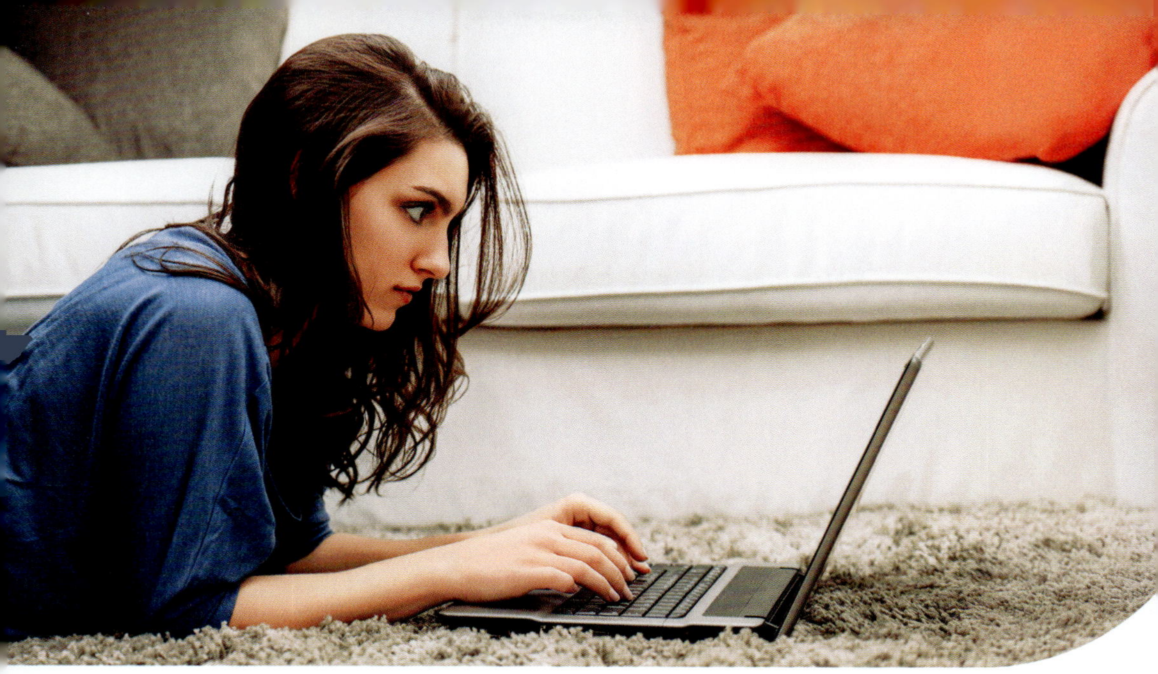

Hyperfocus is not an official symptom of ADHD, and people without ADHD can experience hyperfocus as well.

interested in what she was reading. Soon, she was so focused on the articles that she could not pull herself away. She did well on the quiz and earned a silver medal.

Those with ADHD also tend to be resilient. This means they can bounce back from challenges. They are used to working through difficulties. People with ADHD can also be creative. This can make them great problem solvers. Becca has ADHD.

She explains that it takes her longer to think of ideas. But those ideas are often unique. She finds that people welcome that.

People with ADHD may have a lot of energy. Sometimes this energy can be helpful. Those with ADHD may excel at sports and other activities that require movement. Many professional athletes have been diagnosed with ADHD. They include Olympic swimmer Michael Phelps and Olympic gymnast Simone Biles.

Dr. Ronald Kamm is a sports **psychiatrist**. He says,

> Having ADHD can actually be an advantage in certain sports. You scan the world around you while the coach is talking and take in more than the average kid does. That can

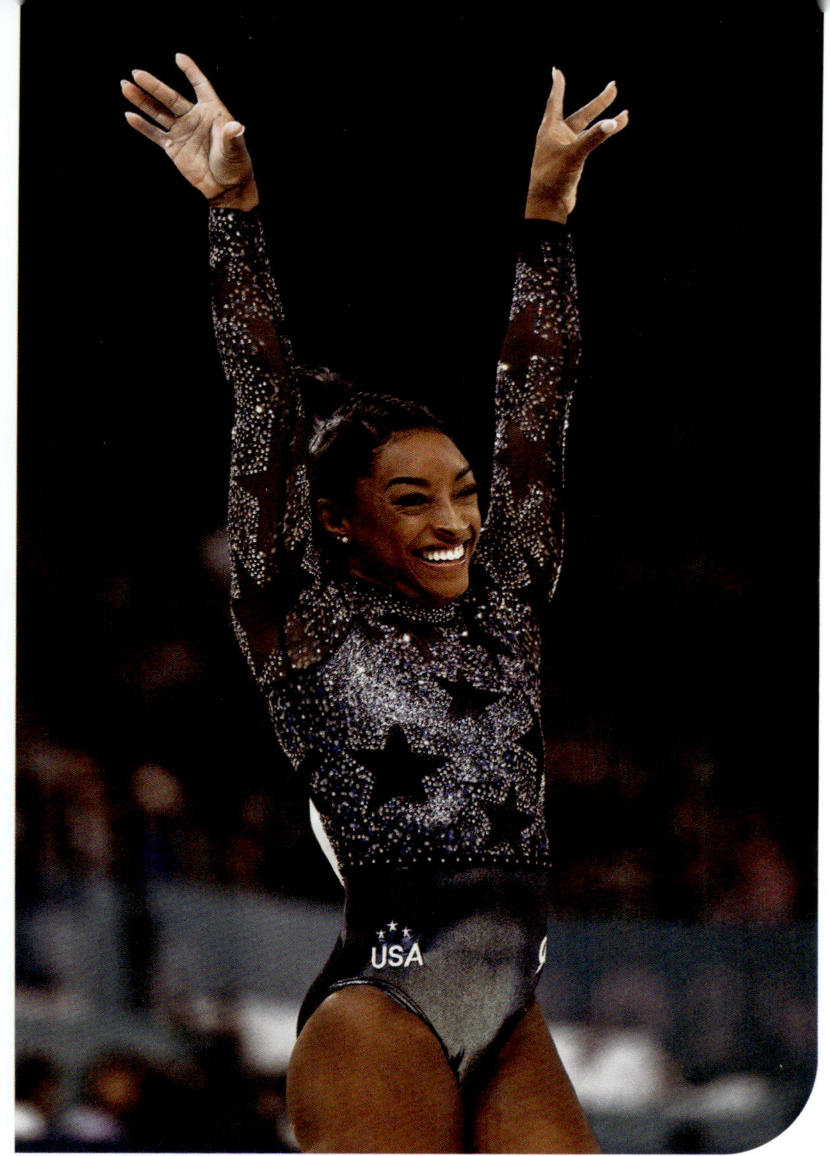



**Simone Biles has said that ADHD is nothing to be ashamed of.**

*work against you in certain situations, like when your mom is talking about cleaning your room. But in athletics it can work for you.*[7]

# FINDING SUPPORT

ADHD diagnoses in US children and teens have risen. They increased from 6 percent in 1997 to about 10 percent in 2016. This has drawn attention to ADHD.

People diagnosed with ADHD are often referred to professionals with ADHD experience. These include counselors, **therapists**, and specialists. Support may be available from parents and teachers. Support groups can help teens with ADHD

**Therapy is not a cure for ADHD. But it may help teens with ADHD cope with the condition.**

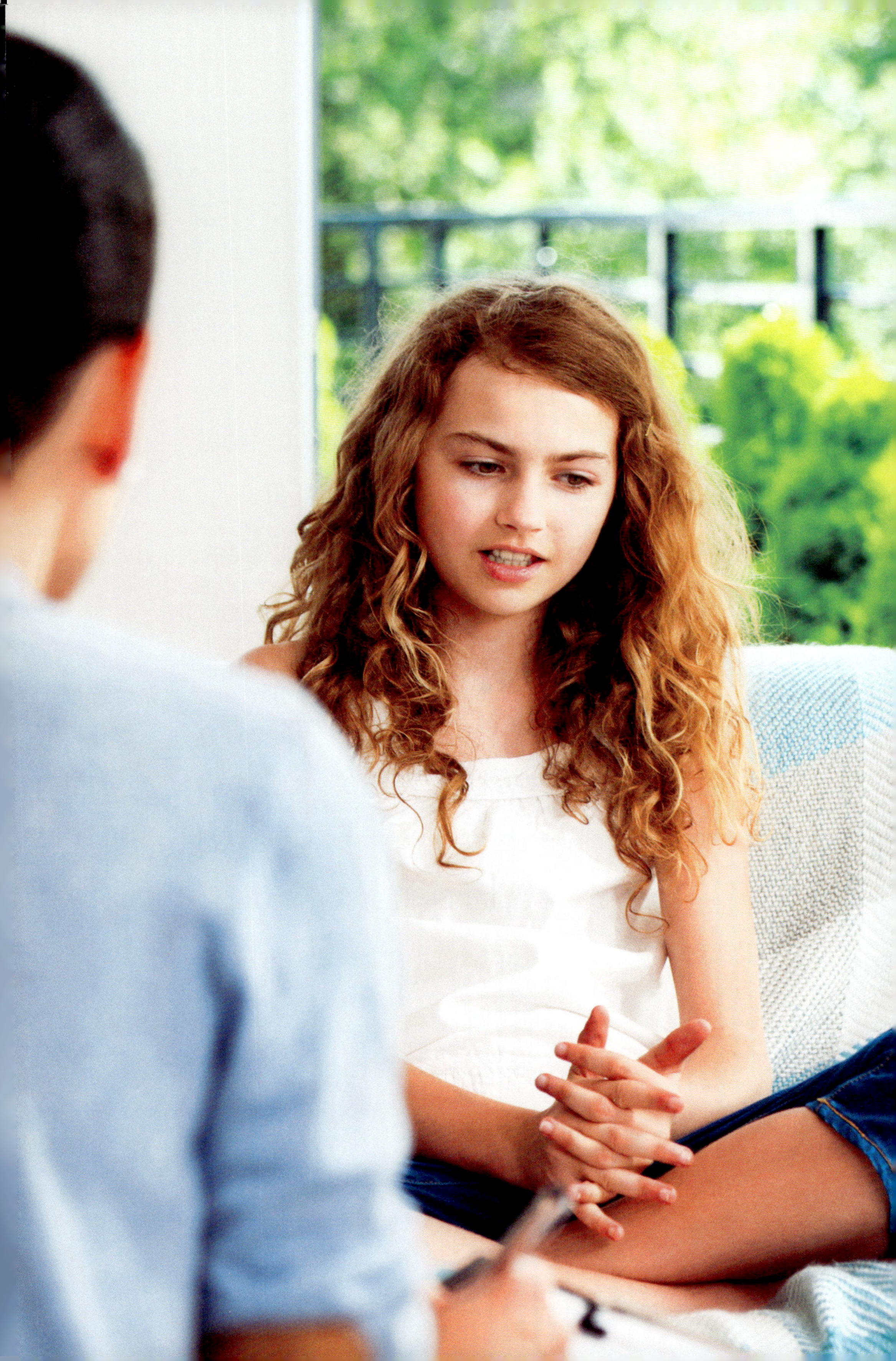

know they are not alone. Medication can also help improve focus.

## THERAPY

Therapy can be an effective way to treat ADHD. Therapists usually meet with patients once per week for at least a few months. They listen as patients talk about how they feel. For therapy to be effective, teens must go to all appointments. They also need to participate in the sessions. Parents or guardians sometimes play a key role. They can help their teen by providing a supportive, structured, and accepting environment at home.

René was 7 years old in 1991 when one professional diagnosed her with ADHD. Doctors did not always support kids with

# WAYS TO NAVIGATE ADHD

- Try new strategies to get organized and see what works for you.

- Make progress on tasks by breaking them into smaller tasks.

- Eat well and get enough sleep and exercise.

- Ask for help when it is needed.

- Stick to an ADHD treatment plan. Take prescribed medication and go to therapy appointments.

- Find solutions to symptoms that work for you.

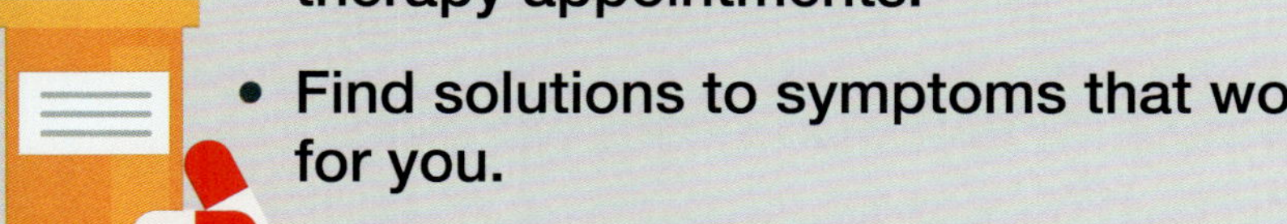

**Many teens with ADHD find success by following some of the strategies above. But each strategy may not work for every teen. Teens with ADHD should follow the guidance of their health care providers.**

ADHD at that time. Black children like René faced additional challenges. René's main doctor ignored her diagnosis. He did not believe in ADHD. René struggled throughout school. She went to college. But she eventually dropped out. She got a job. Soon she was overwhelmed by her work.

René took leave to get better. She went to therapy. René told her therapist she had been diagnosed with ADHD at 7. The therapist immediately referred her to an ADHD specialist. René began to see improvement. "Have you ever switched on a light in a dark room?" she asks. "That's what it felt like once I got my [second] diagnosis. Suddenly I had clarity of mind that I'd never experienced before."[8]

## MEDICATION

Medicine is often used with therapy to treat ADHD symptoms. Medications include stimulants and nonstimulants. Stimulants work by increasing levels

of certain chemicals in the brain.
Nonstimulants help people with ADHD in
other ways.

Both types of medication can be
effective when used under a doctor's care.
Stimulants help 70 to 80 percent of young

To receive ADHD medication, a patient must get a
prescription from a health care professional.

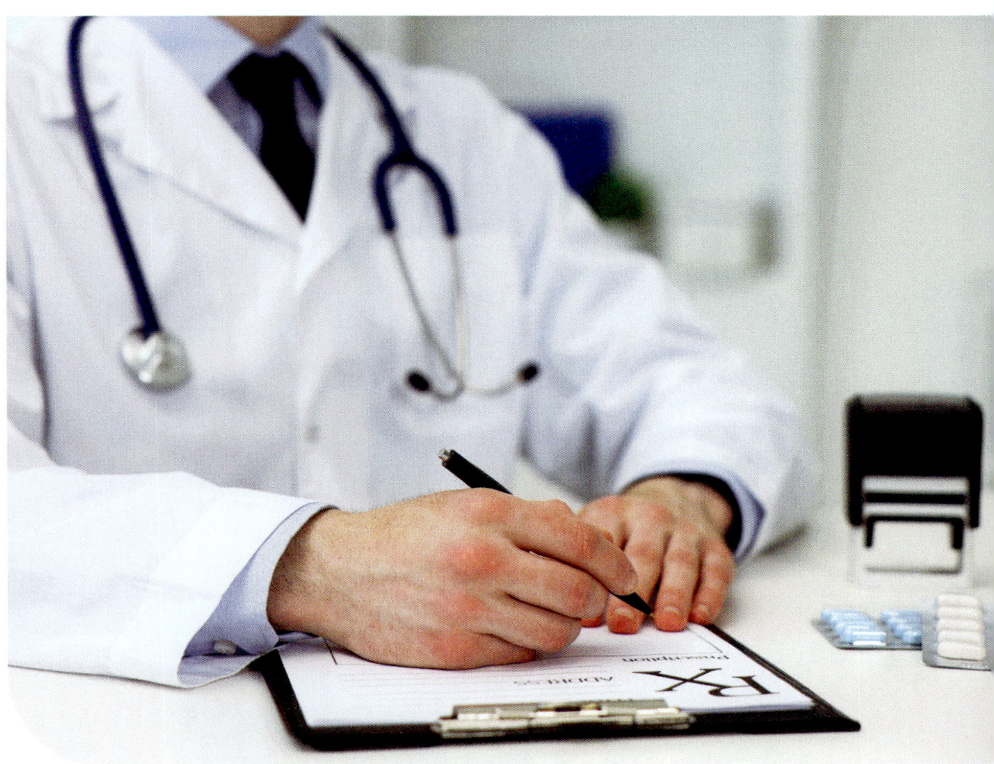

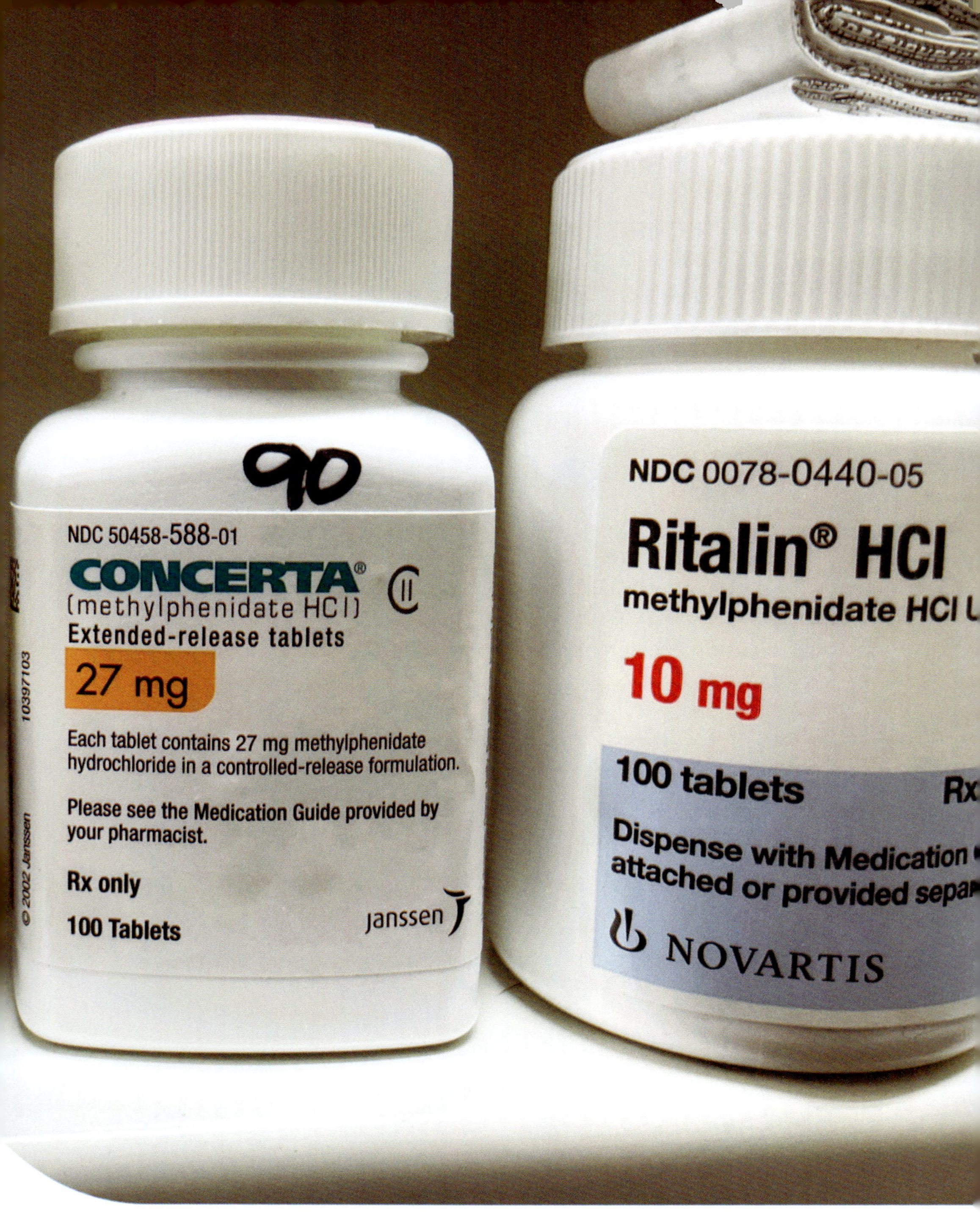


**One of the most commonly prescribed stimulants for ADHD is called Ritalin. However, this medication may not work for everyone.**

people with ADHD have fewer symptoms. Stimulants act quickly. These chemicals help people think and concentrate.

Nonstimulants can also help with ADHD symptoms. They do not act as fast as stimulants. But they do improve symptoms for up to 24 hours. Nonstimulants help people focus and pay attention. They also make people less impulsive.

Jill Dahl had ADHD as a student. She remembers having trouble paying attention in class. Teachers scolded her. Dahl was not diagnosed until she was 29 years old. That was when she started taking medication. She says it changed her life. It allowed her to focus while reading and remember details. She went to college and became a teacher. Now she looks out for her students with ADHD.

Medications can have limited long-term effects. And they may not help improve areas of functioning such as school grades. That is why a combination of medication and therapy is often recommended.

## SUPPORT GROUPS

Support groups can help teens with ADHD. Support groups are gatherings of people who have a shared experience. ADHD support groups welcome people with ADHD and their loved ones. Members of a support group can share their feelings with the group. This can help each member better understand their own experience with ADHD.

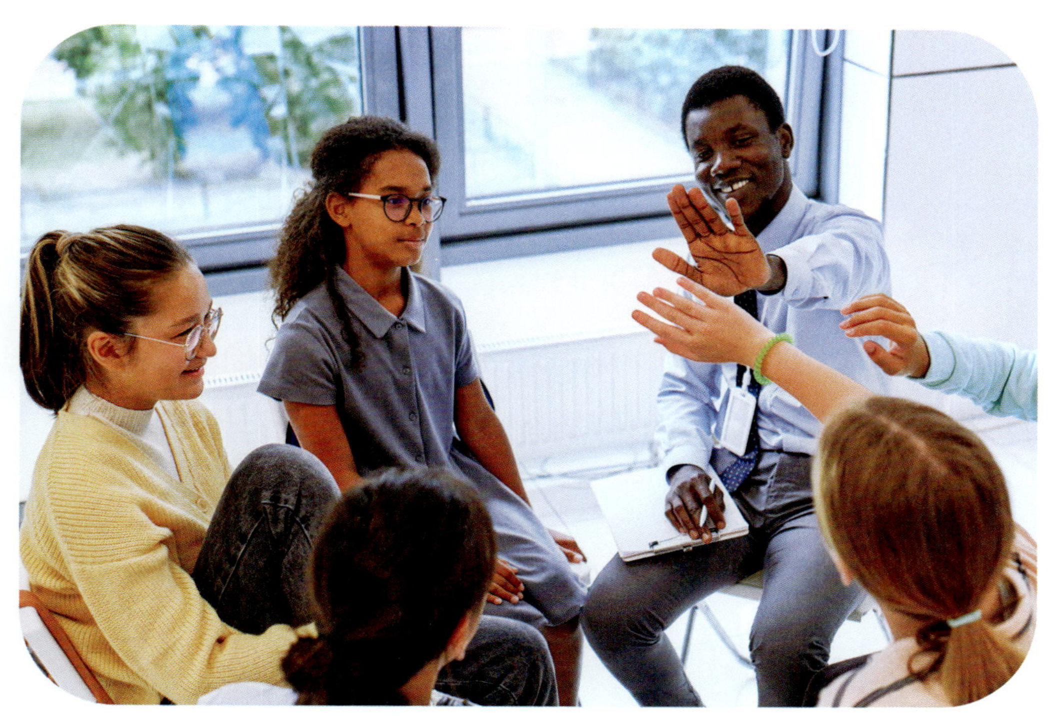

**There are support groups specifically for teens with ADHD.**

Support groups provide emotional support to their members. These meetings let people with ADHD know they are not alone. Dylan found support and acceptance in an online ADHD community. He says, "I am among great people and finally feel like I am not alone. I finally have what I have always deserved regardless of what or how I did something."[9]

Some organizations help people find local or online ADHD support groups. These include Children and Adults with Attention-Deficit/Hyperactivity Disorder (CHADD). Another organization is the Attention Deficit Disorder Association. It holds meetings and other educational events on ADHD. And the Learning

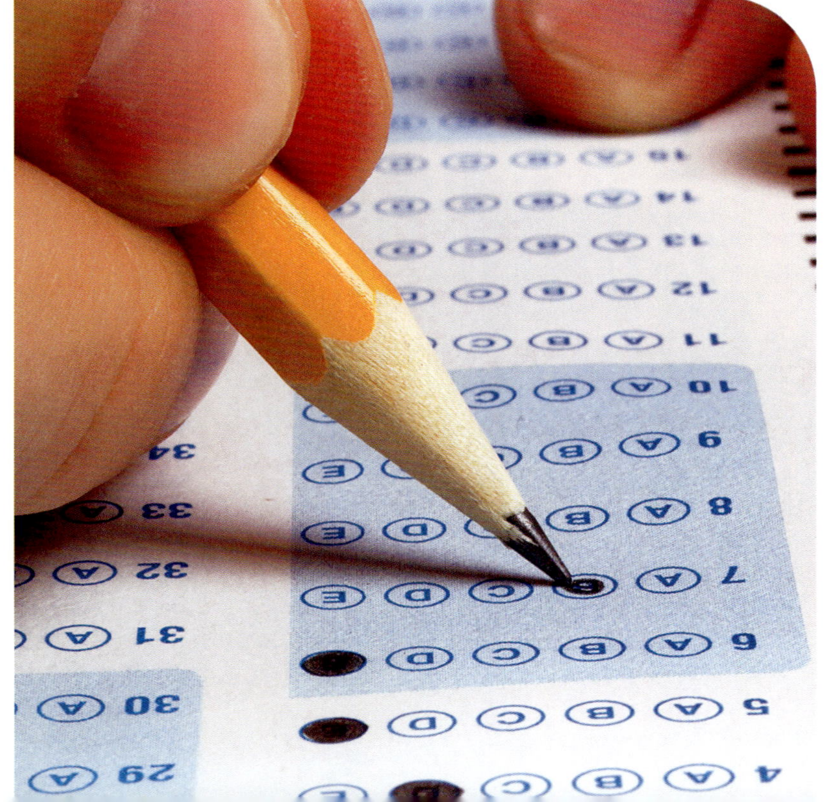

Not every classroom support strategy will help every student with ADHD succeed on tests and classwork.

Disabilities Association of America provides connections to local meetings.

Parents themselves can provide support for their teen with ADHD. Morgan may have never found help for her ADHD symptoms without the support of her mother. Her mother had ADHD herself. She knew her daughter needed help. She **advocated** for Morgan until she got the support she needed.

## CLASSROOM SUPPORT

Students with ADHD have options for support in the classroom. Teachers can make accommodations to help students focus. These may include special seating. This helped Bailey. She was a student with ADHD. She moved to a specific desk in the class for test taking. This helped her focus. Teachers may also give students with ADHD breaks when they need them. And they may work with students to create homework plans.

Some teachers are specially trained to use behavioral classroom management. This means consistently rewarding students for good behavior. This can help students with ADHD. Teaching organizational skills can also help these students. These skills help students learn how to manage their time. They also help students organize their supplies.

Classroom support can make it easier for teens with ADHD to succeed at school. Morgan struggled for most of her early school years with ADHD. Then she enrolled

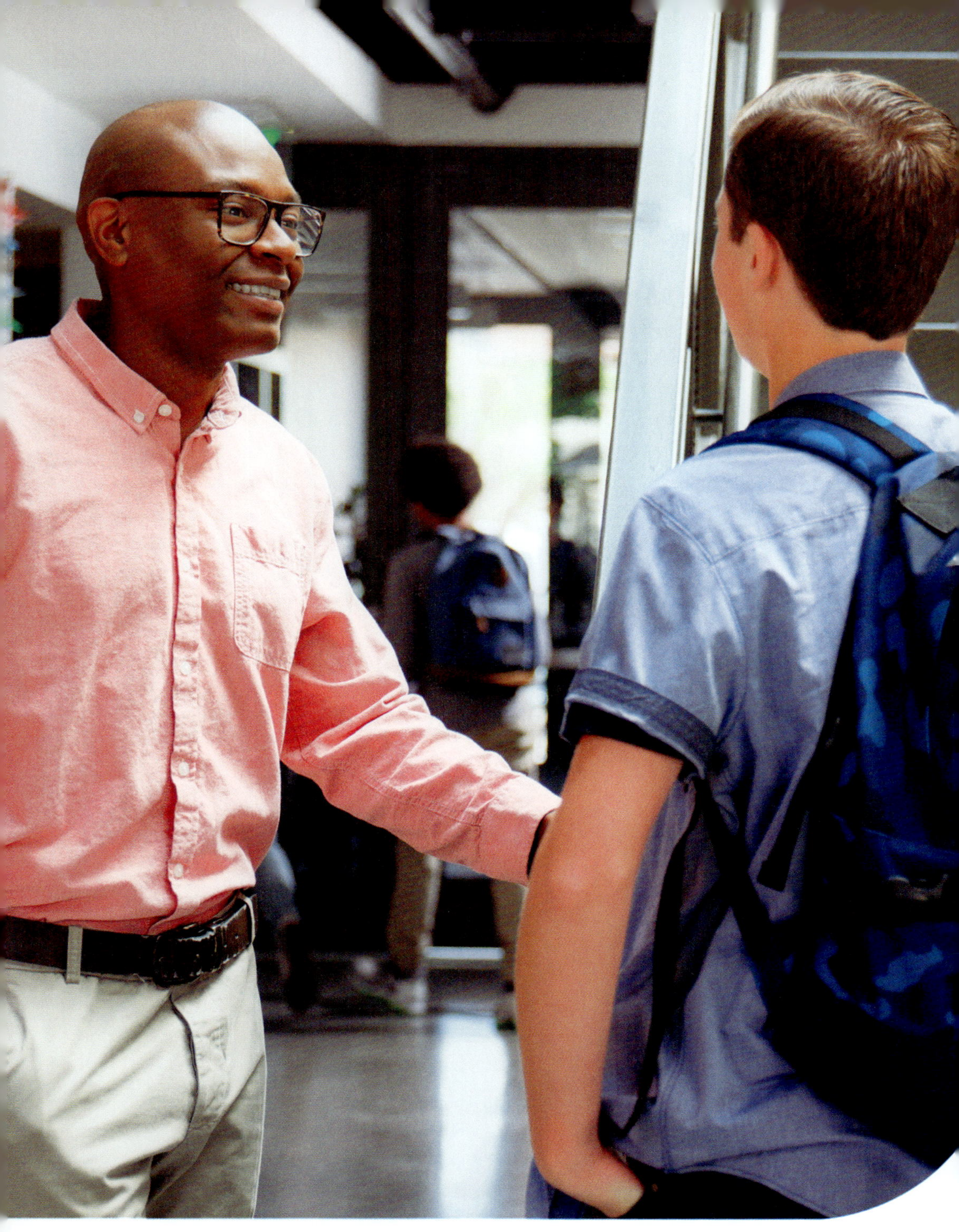

Public schools in the United States have a duty to support students with ADHD.

in a private school for students with learning disabilities such as ADHD. She learned skills to cope with her ADHD. Morgan moved to a big public high school after 4 years. This was a challenge. She still struggled with paying attention. She had to work to listen and remember things. But her social skills and positive attitude helped her succeed.

## Individualized Education Plan

Students with ADHD may receive an individualized education plan (IEP). This document provides specific goals for the student. Each student with an IEP takes a test to determine their learning level. This level is used to create goals for the student. Parents are invited to contribute to this plan based on what they know about how their child learns.

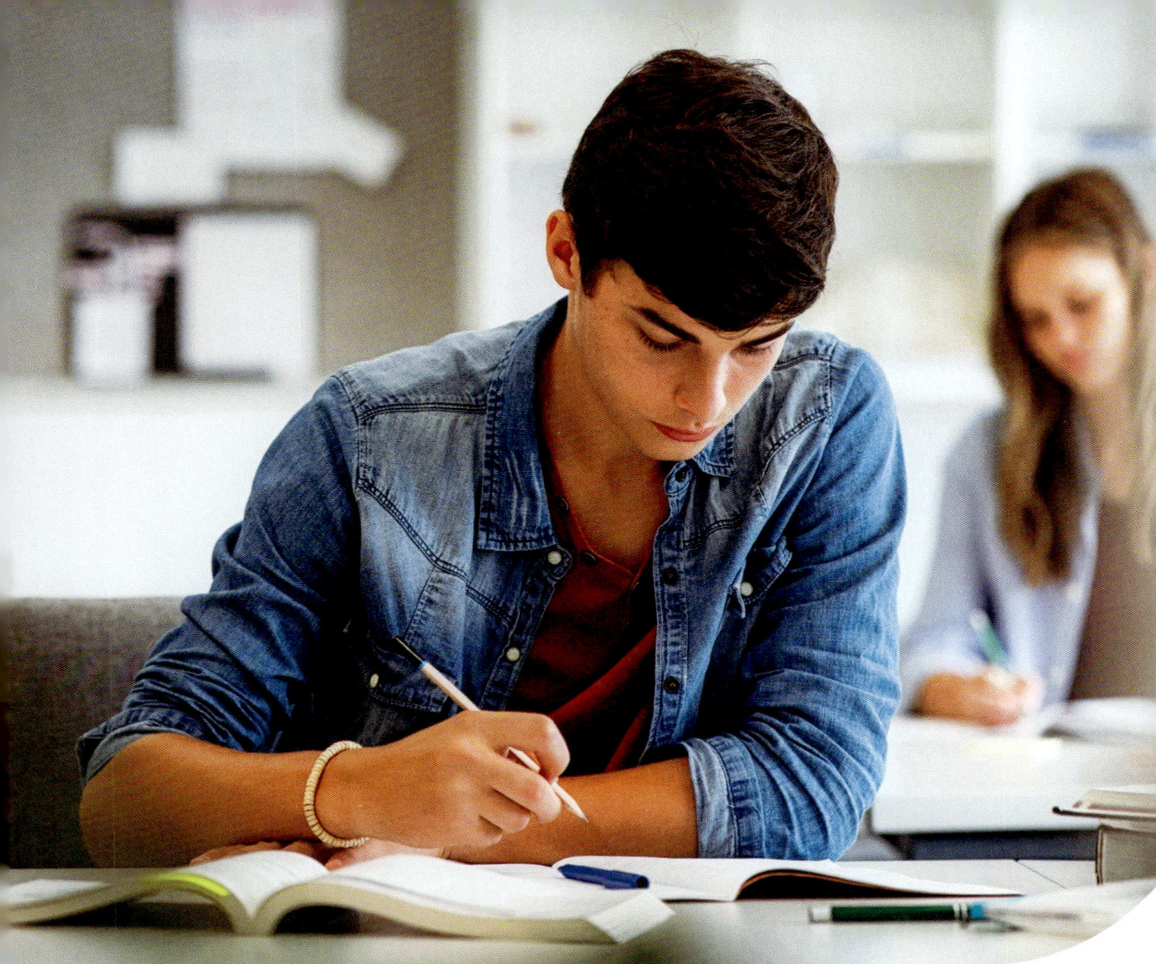



Morgan accepted an award as a 14-year-old for her success in school. She did not know that she would have to give a speech at the event. But she stood in front of more than 350 people and spoke anyway. She thanked those who helped her along the way.

# GLOSSARY

**advocated**
supported a cause or person

**diagnosed**
identified as the cause of symptoms by a medical professional

**medication**
a substance used as a medical treatment

**psychiatrist**
a doctor who treats mental health issues

**psychologist**
a professional who studies how people think, feel, and behave

**self-esteem**
the opinion one has of oneself

**symptoms**
signs of a medical condition

**therapists**
people who treat mental health conditions

### INTRODUCTION: STRUGGLING TO FOCUS

1. Quoted in Keath Low, "A Student's Journey with ADHD," *Attention*, August 2011, pp. 28–30.

### CHAPTER ONE: WHAT IS ADHD?

2. Quoted in "This Is What It's Really Like to Have ADHD," *YouTube*, uploaded by *How to ADHD*, November 16, 2017. www.youtube.com.

### CHAPTER TWO: LIVING WITH ADHD

3. Quoted in "This Is What It's Really Like to Have ADHD."

4. Quoted in "This Is What It's Really Like to Have ADHD."

5. Zoë Kessler, "ADHD: Teen Trouble," *Attention*, April 2014, pp. 24–26.

6. Quoted in Gina Pera, "One Man's Story: Growing Up Undiagnosed ADHD," *ADHD Roller Coaster*, May 30, 2018. https://adhdrollercoaster.org.

7. Quoted in Aimee Crawford, "Bravo, Simone Biles, for Taking a Stand Against ADHD Stigma," *ESPN*, September 21, 2016. www.espn.com.

### CHAPTER THREE: FINDING SUPPORT

8. René Brooks, "How a Late ADHD Diagnosis Changed My Life," *Teva*, May 16, 2018. www.tevapharm.com.

9. Quoted in Pera, "One Man's Story: Growing Up Undiagnosed ADHD."

## BOOKS

Mary Bates, *Teen Guide: Depression*. BrightPoint Press, 2026.

Tammy Gagne, *Teens Dealing with Learning Disorders*. BrightPoint Press, 2025.

Alice Gendron, *The Mini ADHD Coach*. Chronicle Prism, 2023.

## INTERNET SOURCES

"ADHD Information for Teens," *CHADD*, n.d. https://chadd.org.

"Data and Statistics on ADHD," *Centers for Disease Control and Prevention*, May 16, 2024. www.cdc.gov.

"What Is ADHD?" *Nemours Teens Health*, May 2022. https://kidshealth.org.

# WEBSITES

## Attention Deficit Disorder Association (ADDA)
https://add.org

The Attention Deficit Disorder Association is a nonprofit organization dedicated to providing resources to help those with ADHD. It publishes a monthly newsletter and connects people with peer support groups.

## Children and Adults with Attention Deficit/ Hyperactivity Disorder (CHADD)
https://chadd.org

The Children and Adults with Attention Deficit/Hyperactivity Disorder website provides a source for information about ADHD. It supports those with ADHD and their families, providing the tools and education they need to successfully navigate life with ADHD.

## Learning Disabilities Association of America
www.ldaamerica.org

The Learning Disabilities Association of America works to advocate for people with learning disabilities. Its website contains educational material for parents and teachers, as well as resources for people with learning disabilities.

# INDEX

# IMAGE CREDITS

Cover: © Antonio Guillem/Shutterstock Images

5: © fizkes/Shutterstock Images

7: © PeopleImages.com-Yuri A./Shutterstock Images

8: © Drazen Zigic/Shutterstock Images

10: © Take A Pix Media/Shutterstock Images

13: © sirtravelalot/Shutterstock Images

14: © carballo/Shutterstock Images

17: © MDV Edwards/Shutterstock Images

18: © illustrissima/Shutterstock Images

20: © fizkes/Shutterstock Images

22: © Ground Picture/Shutterstock Images

24: © New Africa/Shutterstock Images

25: © Suzanne Tucker/Shutterstock Images

27: © Joko P./Shutterstock Images

29: © Asian Isolated/Shutterstock Images

30: © PeopleImages.com-Yuri A./Shutterstock Images

34: © fizkes/Shutterstock Images

36: © Christy Thompson/Shutterstock Images

37: © Asia Images Group/Shutterstock Images

39: © Giulio_Fornasar/Shutterstock Images

41: © A. Ricardo/Shutterstock Images

43: © izusek/iStockphoto

45 (checklist): © Aleksandr_Lysenko/Shutterstock Images

45 (bed): © Mary Long/Shutterstock Images

45 (medicine): © Danielala/Shutterstock Images

47: © New Africa/Shutterstock Images

48: © PureRadiancePhoto/Shutterstock Images

51: © SeventyFour/Shutterstock Images

52: © Constantine Pankin/Shutterstock Images

55: © Monkey Business Images/Shutterstock Images

57: © Ground Picture/Shutterstock Images

Kari A. Cornell is an award-winning author of books for young people. She gardens, runs, and makes pottery. She lives in Minneapolis with her husband, two boys, and their sweet dog, EmmyLou.